The Complete Ketogenic Diet for Beginners 2021.

Mary Perry

Index

Sommario

Ketogenic diet an introduction

The word "Ketogenic" means a diet with low-carb content (like the Atkins diet). In this type of diet, body gets calories from proteins and fats instead of carbohydrates.

This is very low carb and high fats diet and is a lot similar to Atkins and other low carb diets. The main idea of ketogenic diet is to reduce the intake of carbohydrates and replace most of the carbs with fats. This reduction in carbohydrates intake starts a metabolic activity called "ketosis" in the body. This diet got its name by this "ketosis" process.

In this metabolic state, the body efficiently burns fat for energy. It is also good for brain as it also converts fat into ketones in lever that transfer energy to brain.

In ketogenic diet, the foods we mostly eat contain 55% to 60% fat, 30% to 35% protein and 5% to 10% carbohydrates.

Origin of ketogenic diet:

Historically speaking, Russell Wilder in 1921 first used the ketogenic diet to treat epilepsy. For more than 10 years the ketogenic diet was used as a medical treatment for pediatric epilepsy. But with the passage of time, the idea started to build to use the ketogenic diet as a rapid weight loss formula. In present days, ketogenic diet is more popular as a weight losing formula as compared to a medical treatment. But yes! Weight loss is not less than a medical treatment as well.

Types of ketogenic diet

Ketogenic diet evolved through medical and scientific processes. The experts have categorized the ketogenic diet into 4 types.

1-Standard Ketogenic diet (SKD) :

This is a high fat diet with moderate protein content and very low carb content. It contains 70 % fat, 20 % protein and 10 % carbs.

2-Cyclical ketogenic diet (CKD):

This is a periodic type diet plan. It comprises of periods of low carb fee and high carb refeeds. For example, a 7-day cyclical diet plan means 5 days ketogenic days with low carb intake followed by 2 days with high carb intake.

3-Targeted ketogenic diet (TKD):

This diet allows you to add carbs during workout or exercise.

4-High protein ketogenic diet:

Just like standard ketogenic diet, this is low carb diet. But protein content is more than SKD. The ratio is often 60 % fat, 35 % protein and 5 % carbs.

However, only the standard and high protein ketogenic diets have been studied comprehensively. The other two types are considered more advanced methods and are used by body builders or athletes etc.

Health Benefits of ketogenic diet: A tasty medicine

Weight loss:

The medical sciences have advanced a lot but there still remain some challenges. Obesity is one of the greatest challenges that stand in front of the medical sciences. Obesity continue to remain a worldwide health problem and a challenge with adult mortality as high as 2.8 million per year. Obesity is not a single disease but it invites a lot of other chronic diseases as well. The diseases like diabetes, hypertension and heart diseases are largely related to obesity. Obesity is mainly caused due to unhealthy life style and poor dietary habits and routines.

Ketogenic diet has brought a hope for people suffering from obesity. It is for sure not the ultimate cure for the disease but can reduce the weight up to a large extent. And if an individual puts some more effort than surely this diet can be proven as the desired cure for the obesity.

The prime purpose and benefit of ketogenic diet is weight loss. Studies found that ketogenic diet was more effective than a low-fat diet for weight loss. But ketogenic diet is not confined to just weight loss; there are other health benefits as well.

Studies found that people following ketogenic diet are less exposed to diabetes or pre-diabetes. Keto diet boosts the insulin sensitivity and burns fat. It is also found that type 2 diabetic patients have decreased level of diabetes after following ketogenic diet. Ketogenic diet causes reduction in seizures in epilepsy. It is also beneficial and is kinds of tasty cure for heart diseases, cancer, Parkinson's disease, polycystic ovary syndrome and brain diseases.

The science of ketogenic diet

How does keto diet work?

Basically, carbohydrates are the primary source of energy production in body tissues. When the body is deprived of carbohydrates due to reducing intake to less than 50g per day, insulin secretion is significantly reduced and the body enters a catabolic state. Glycogen stores deplete, forcing the body to go through certain metabolic changes. Two metabolic processes come into action when there is low carbohydrate availability in body tissues: gluconeogenesis and ketogenesis.

Gluconeogenesis is the endogenous production of glucose in the body, especially in the liver primarily from lactic acid, glycerol, and the amino acids alanine and glutamine. When glucose availability drops further, the endogenous production of glucose is not able to keep up with the needs of the body and ketogenesis begins in order to provide an alternate source of energy in the form of ketone bodies. Ketone bodies replace glucose as a primary source of energy. During ketogenesis due to low blood glucose feedback, stimulus for insulin secretion is also low, which sharply reduces the stimulus for fat and glucose storage. Other hormonal changes may contribute to the increased breakdown of fats that result in fatty acids. Fatty acids are metabolized to acetoacetate which is later converted to beta-hydroxybutyrate and acetone. These are the basic ketone bodies that accumulate in the body as a ketogenic diet is sustained. This metabolic state is referred to as "nutritional ketosis." As long as the body is deprived of carbohydrates, metabolism remains in the ketotic state. The nutritional ketosis state is considered quite safe, as ketone bodies are produced in small concentrations without any alterations in blood pH. It greatly differs from ketoacidosis, a life-threatening condition where ketone bodies are produced in extremely larger concentrations, altering blood pH to acidotic a state.

Ketone bodies synthesized in the body can be easily utilized for energy production by heart, muscle tissue, and the kidneys. Ketone bodies also can cross the blood-brain barrier to provide an alternative source of energy to the brain. RBCs and the liver do not utilize ketones due to lack of mitochondria and enzyme diaphoresis respectively. Ketone body production depends on several factors such as resting basal metabolic rate (BMR), body mass index (BMI), and body fat percentage. One hundred grams of acetoacetate generates 9400 grams of ATP, and 100 g of beta-hydroxybutyrate yields 10,500 grams of ATP; whereas, 100 grams of glucose produces only 8,700 grams of ATP. This allows the body to maintain efficient fuel production even during a caloric deficit. Ketone bodies also decrease free radical damage and enhance antioxidant capacity.

Summary:

On a simple and short note, ketogenic diet works as an alternative of glucose. Human body experiences two processes to get energy. First is gluconeogenesis, in this process body tissues and muscles use glucose as a source which is mainly produced in the liver. When carbs intake is reduced the production of glucose decreases. As a result, body starts finding an alternative to get energy. It is the time when another process 'ketogenesis' starts. In ketogenesis, body starts getting energy from fats and as a result body fat burns and man starts losing weight.

Important questions and their answers

1-Who can and cannot follow the keto diet?

It is not necessary that only people suffering from obesity can follow the keto diet, this diet for everyone as it is healthier and energetic. So, anyone who is willing can follow the diet.

Yet there are some people who cannot follow the ketogenic diet plan because of some diseases. People suffering from diabetes and taking insulin or oral hypoglycemic agents suffer severe hypoglycemia if the medications are not appropriately adjusted before initiating this diet. The ketogenic diet is contraindicated in patients with pancreatitis, liver failure, disorders of fat metabolism, primary carnitine deficiency, carnitine palmitoyl transferase deficiency, carnitine translocase deficiency, porphyria, or pyruvate kinase deficiency. People on a ketogenic diet rarely can have a false positive breath alcohol test. Due to ketonemia, acetone in the body can sometimes be reduced to isopropanol by hepatic alcohol dehydrogenase which can give a false positive alcohol breath test result.

2-Does it cost too much to follow ketogenic diet?

Well, that's not a case. Even if it cost a bit, would you ignore its medicinal benefits? But still it doesn't cost any extra money and, in some cases, it is less expensive than normal day diets. Moreover, it saves your pocket because you stop spending your earnings on fast foods and junk foods. You also leave most of the cold drinks and juices that are high carb and as a result this diet proves to be a very budget friendly and even a budget helping diet.

The ingredients and tools that are mostly used to prepare ketogenic meal are less expensive and are mostly available at home or local market. Most of the vegetables used are not so expensive. Sometimes you need to use olive oil or avocado oil for cooking and frying purposes, these types of ingredients may cost you a little. Use of mozzarella cheese and cream cheese also adds up in cost and often makes the diet expensive but still, one is not going to eat cheesy meal daily so you need not to worry about the cost. It is completely budget friendly and, in some cases, if it is costly, then remember its health benefits.

The recipes that are discussed in this book are moderate. There are some recipes that may be a little costly but there are also some recipes that will not cost you a lot. So, this book is a complete package containing basic, standard and premier recipes so that people may decide to choose a recipe according to their pocket.

3-Is it harmful for body?

It is not harmful for body if is done within limits prescribed by medical experts. It is universal truth that excess of anything is poisonous. Same is the matter in this case. If ketogenic diets are taken for a much longer time, the glucose will decrease to a vulnerable amount in body. As a result, the ketogenesis will start increasing acidity in the blood. That's why it is advised to follow ketogenic diet in form of a short-term plan.

4-What to eat and what avoid during keto diet:

So that is the most common question that comes in minds of most of the people while talking about ketogenic diet. Everyone doesn't have a laboratory at home to test which ingredients are high carb and which one is low carb. So, let's see, what things we have to avoid during the keto diet.

First of all, forget the fast and junk food! You cannot go near to it if you are following a keto plan.

Secondly, consider the drinks your worst enemies. The drinks are one of the biggest causes of obesity worldwide. So, keep yourself away from this poison.

Thirdly, you will need to leave few things that you love a lot, surely you are not going to leave your wife or husband but yes! You will need to leave bread, sugar, starches and sometimes potatoes also. It means no more fries, no more crispy potato chips. But you've got some best dishes in ketogenic menu that will make you forget fries and fast food. So, you need not to worry much!

One more a vastly used thing that you are going to leave is cooked rice. But there is an alternative for it. You can enjoy the taste of rice in shape of cauliflower rice and the cauliflower recipes are also included in the recipe list.

Other than these, you can use almost all the ingredients you like.

So, that was all about understanding ketogenic diet. Now! It's time to start following and preparing the diet in a delicious way. Let's get into the kitchen of keto diet and reduce weight with a tasty medicine!

FOODS TO ENJOY ON THE KETOGENIC DIET

There are different types of food that fall into this list. These food ideas definitely push for high fat content, while at the same time packing other nutrients and healthy vitamins in for the body's use.

Meats And Animal Products – Focus on grass-fed or pasture-raised fatty cuts of meat and wild-caught seafood, avoiding farmed animal meats and processed meats as much as possible. And don't forget about organ meats!

- Beef
- Chicken
- Eggs
- Goat
- Lamb
- Pork
- Rabbit
- Turkey
- Venison
- Shellfish
- Salmon
- Mackerel
- Tuna
- Halibut
- Cod
- Gelatin
- Organ meats

Healthy Fats – The best fats to consume on the ketogenic diet are monounsaturated and polyunsaturated fats, though there are plenty of healthy saturated fats as well. At the risk of sounding like a broken recorder, avoid Trans fats. Maybe "avoid" is not an appropriate word. Run away might be better. Run away from Trans fats like you would the plague. Enough said.

- o Butter
- o Chicken fat
- o Coconut oil
- o Duck fat
- o Ghee
- o Lard
- o Tallow
- o MCT oil
- o Avocado oil
- o Macadamia oil
- o Extra virgin olive oil
- o Coconut butter
- o Coconut milk
- o Palm shortening

Vegetables – Fresh vegetables are rich in nutrients and low in calories which make them an excellent addition to any diet.

- o Artichokes
- o Asparagus
- o Avocado
- o Bell peppers
- o Broccoli

- Cabbage
- Cauliflower
- Cucumber
- Celery
- Kohlrabi
- Lettuce
- Okra or ladies' fingers
- Radishes
- Seaweed
- Spinach
- Tomatoes
- Watercress
- Zucchini

Dairy Products – **If you are able to tolerate dairy, you can include full-fat, unpasteurized, and raw dairy products in your diet. Keep in mind that some brands will contain a lot of sugar which could increase the carb content, so pay attention to nutrition labels and moderate your consumption of these products. If possible, go for the full-fat versions as these will have a less likely chance of sugar being used to replace the fat.**

- Kefir
- Cottage cheese
- Cream cheese
- Cheddar cheese
- Brie cheese
- Mozzarella cheese
- Swiss cheese
- Sour cream

- o Full-fat yogurt
- o Heavy cream

Herbs And Spices – Fresh herbs and dried spices are an excellent way to flavor your foods without adding any significant number of calories or carbohydrates

- o Basil
- o Black pepper
- o Cayenne
- o Cardamom
- o Chili powder
- o Cilantro
- o Cinnamon
- o Cumin
- o Curry powder
- o Garam masala
- o Ginger
- o Garlic
- o Nutmeg
- o Oregano
- o Onion
- o Paprika
- o Parsley
- o Rosemary
- o Sea salt
- o Sage
- o Thyme
- o Turmeric
- o White pepper

Beverages – You should avoid all sweetened drinks on the ketogenic diet, but there are certain beverages which you can still have in order to add a little more variety to your choice of liquids besides good old water.

- Almond milk unsweetened
- Bone broth
- Cashew milk unsweetened
- Coconut milk
- Club soda
- Coffee
- Herbal tea
- Mineral water
- Seltzer water
- Tea

FOODS ON THE MODERATION LIST

These food items are included here because they tend to have a higher carb count, so moderation is important. However, they are chocking full of other nutrients and some of them also throw in that extra bit of fat to help toward your daily fat intake! Fruits – Fresh fruits are an excellent source of nutrition. Unfortunately, they are also loaded with sugar which means they are high in carbohydrates. There are a few low- to moderate-carb fruits that you can enjoy in smaller quantities, but you have to watch the amount you eat! Sometimes, it is really easy to keep popping them into our mouths. "Nature's candy" is definitely an accurate moniker for them. We can still get their benefits and maintain ketosis with the right amounts of consumption. Most of the fruits detailed below are okay for you to have a cup or so, perhaps a single slice or two on a daily basis, especially when you are first starting out and are looking to keep your carb count low. As you progress and get a better handle of your carb threshold, it is alright to increase the quantity of these foods while staying within your designated carb limit.

- Apricot
- Blackberries
- Blueberries
- Cantaloupe
- Cherries
- Cranberries
- Grapefruit
- Honeydew
- Kiwi
- Lemon
- Lime
- Peaches
- Raspberries
- Strawberries

Nuts And Seeds – While nuts and seeds do contain carbohydrates, they are also rich in healthy fats. The following nuts and seeds are low to moderate in carb content, so you can enjoy them as long as you watch your portion sizes. Usually an ounce or a handful of nuts would be a good gauge to see how much you can eat and still stay in ketosis daily.

- Almonds

- Cashews
- Chia seeds
- Hazelnuts
- Macadamia nuts
- Pecans
- Pine nuts
- Pistachios
- Psyllium
- Pumpkin seeds
- Sesame seeds
- Sunflower seeds
- Walnuts
- Nut butter

Here is a quick list of some of the major foods you'll need to avoid on the ketogenic diet.

- All-purpose flour
- Baking mix
- Wheat flour
- Pastry flour
- Cake flour
- Cereal
- Pasta
- Rice
- Corn
- Baked goods
- Corn syrup
- Snack bars
- Quinoa
- Buckwheat

- Barley
- Couscous
- Oats
- Muesli
- Margarine
- Canola oil
- Hydrogenated oils
- Bananas
- Mangos
- Pineapple
- Potatoes
- Sweet potatoes
- Candy
- Milk chocolate
- Ice cream
- Sports drinks
- Juice cocktail
- Soda
- Beer
- Milk
- Low-fat dairy
- White sugar
- Brown sugar
- Maple syrup
- Honey
- Agave

WHAT TO LOOK OUT FOR IN SOME KETO FOODS

Since this is very much serving as a recipe book, I thought it would be appropriate to share some tips and ideas on what to look out for when we are choosing the more common and popular keto foods for prepping our meals.

Salmon – This fatty fish has always ranked high for me when it comes to keto friendly foods. You may know it to be packed with beneficial omega-3 polyunsaturated fats, which boost brain health and help with reducing inflammation, but it also has loads of other nutrients which the body needs. Potassium and selenium are found in bountiful amounts when it comes to salmon. Potassium is integral to proper regulation of blood pressure as well as the body's water retention. Selenium helps out with maintaining good bone health as well as ensuring an optimal immune system. On top of this, salmon also contains healthy levels of B vitamins. These vitamins are crucial for efficient food to energy processing, as well as maintaining the proper function of both the body's DNA and nervous system. To top it off, salmon has astaxanthin, an antioxidant which gives salmon flesh its reddish-pink hue. This powerful antioxidant helps with heart and brain health, and may also be beneficial for the skin. To get a good quality deal, the first thing you should take note of is the smell. Fresh salmon, or any fish for that matter, will not really have an odor. You can probably smell a tinge of the ocean, but fresh fish will definitely not smell fishy. When it is fishy, you know that fish is not for you. Next up, pay attention to the eyes. Look for those with clear and shiny eyes. Think of a movie star who has teared up - those are the kind of eyes that best demonstrate what you are looking for. Never go for sunken or dry-looking eyes. Cloudy-looking ones are also a no-go when it comes to fresh fish selection. Fins and gills are also areas which we want to pay attention to. Fresh fish have fins which look wet and whole, not torn and ragged. Their gills are bright red and clean, not brownish-red and slimy. Lastly, if you are allowed to, try pressing the flesh and seeing if it bounces back like how your own does. Flesh which is depressed and stays depressed should not end up in your kitchen. For fillet cuts, the best you can do is pay attention to the color as well as how the piece looks. The color should be vibrant and bright. Varied hues ranging from red to coral to pink are acceptable, but always remember that the main thing is the brightness of the flesh. Next would be to spot any breaks or cracks in the flesh itself. These are indications that the fillet has been kept for some time and is no longer as fresh. Also, any pooling of water should also trigger alarm bells, because it means that the flesh structure has started to break down, and it is time to move on to another piece.

Pork belly – This is another probable staple in the keto diet. I've talked about it in my other book but here I want to concentrate on helping you choose a good cut for prepping your meals. Every 100 grams of pork belly contains about 50 grams of fat. Packing another 9 grams of protein and absolutely no carbs, you can be sure that this is a good food item to boost your daily fat count. On top of that, it can be absolutely easy to prepare delicious meals with it. When choosing pork belly, you should look at the color of the cut. Go for the cuts that are reddish pink to darkish red. Meat which is lighter in color generally means the freshness may have faded. Greying or discoloration will definitely mean that decay has already set in and the meat should not be picked up. The other thing you want to look for is the streaky white strips of fat present in the pork belly. Generally the more streaks it has, the better the marbling will be and that is good news for you. Always ensure that the marbling is white, because any yellow or greyish coloring would represent meat that has probably passed its sell-by date.

Avocado oil – I must be honest here and say that this oil, for me, has been a later stage addition when compared to olive and coconut oil. Extra virgin olive oil, as well as the versatile coconut oil have their rightful places in the pantheon of staple keto foods, but avocado oil might be giving them a run for their money. Avocado oil for one, consists of mostly monounsaturated fat. This particular quirk ties in to a very important point. The oil is considered far more stable than any of its polyunsaturated fat cousins, like vegetable oil and even extra virgin olive oil. Besides that, avocado oil is known to have a higher smoke point, somewhere around 500 degrees Fahrenheit, than most vegetable oils. This makes it a valuable addition to the kitchen because the oil has a higher vitamins, minerals, phytochemicals, and antioxidants, you will realize that this is one oil you can potentially use for many different applications. Some folks use it for hair and skin care, where the vitamin E rich oil is known to be easily absorbed without additional chemicals or other potentially harmful additives. Adding the oil into salads, vegetables, or fruits is also a great way to boost monounsaturated fat intake with very little inconvenience. You might even want to try drinking it raw, though it doesn't work for me as I found it to be a little too raw. Mixing it up with some lime or garlic has always been what I prefer. Now let's talk a little on how to go about choosing the avocado oil. First up, we want to look at the source or origin of the oil, which typically means we need to know where and how the avocados were grown. In this respect, you need to look for a certified organic label to know that the avocados were grown without any synthetic additives. This ensures that the oil derived from the avocados do not contain any substances that could be detrimental to your health. Next, we need to look at how the oil is extracted. Mechanical and chemical extraction methods used usually involves increased heat as well as potent chemicals to force out the oil from the mashed avocado pulp. The downside of this is that the heat and chemicals may reduce the beneficial nutrients and vitamins present in the oil. To address this, cold pressing, which is known as the least destructive method out there, ensures that the color, smell, and taste are as close to the original fruit as possible. You get better quality oil, and in addition to that, enjoy more nutrients. The last item we need to look at is how the oil is refined, or not. Seriously, for best results, cold pressed oil that is unrefined and gotten from certified organic avocados, would rank amongst the top tiers, if not the top. That shouldn't be a problem if you use it often, and you should, considering the health benefits and convenience that it brings. The next best thing would be to have the oil naturally refined, where the manufacturers typically do straining and filtering in order to extend the shelf life. Always remember, the more the oil is refined, the less nutrition it will provide. Before I forget, always opt for oils in dark-colored glass bottles or tins. This is a little similar to extra virgin olive oil where the oil can go rancid in the presence of heat and light. For avocado oil, though the majority of fats present consist of the monounsaturated variety, there still is a minor percentage of polyunsaturated fats. Hence, better to err on the side of caution and go for dark-colored glass bottles.

RECIPES

Low carb rice (cauliflower rice):

Cauliflower rice itself is a simple dish but it opens doors to a whole heaven of toppings and variations that you can try on it. It can bear any kind of topping and that is beauty of this dish. You can add cream cheese, mint leaves, mint sauce, red chili sauce, seasoned tacos, mushrooms, vegetables, beans, peanuts, almond, walnut and a lot more as toppings. You just need to imagine and be creative, then see the magical taste and look of this dish. It is going to be the delicious meal today!

Time required:

15 minutes, ready to serve in 30 minutes

Ingredients:

- o Cauliflower florets – 8 cups
- o Olive oil – 3 tsp
- o Mozzarella smoked and chopped – 4 ounces
- o Roasted red pepper – 6 ounces

- Banana pepper rings -1 ounce
- Sliced olives – ½ cup
- Basil chopped – 1 cup
- Vinegar – 3 tsp
- Salt and pepper to taste

Instructions:

- Pre-heat oven to 370-400°F. Place cauliflower florets on baking pan and add olive oil into it.
- Bake for 50-60 minutes then place the baked cauliflower florets into a food processor and pulse until texture of rice.
- Now cook the cauliflower rice in a large skillet tossing with the olive oil until warmed and then follow the rest of recipe.
- Now pour the rice into a bowl and allow to cool.
- Once cooled, add other remaining ingredients into the bowl and mix together. Sprinkle salt and pepper to taste and enjoy the dish.

Ketogenic stuffed mushrooms:

The simple yet versatile dish. You are going to love this.

Time required:

20 minutes, ready to serve in 40 minutes

Ingredients:

- Mushrooms – 12
- Bacon – 8 oz
- Butter – 2 tsp
- Cream cheese – 9 oz
- Paprika powder – 1 tsp
- Finely chopped – 3tsp
- Butter – 2 tsp
- Salt and pepper to taste

Instructions:

- Preheat the oven to 400°F (200°C). Take a baking dish and grease it with butter.
- Take a pan and put over medium heat. Fry the bacon in the pan until crispy. Let cool and crush into crumbs. Save the bacon fat.
- Remove the mushroom stems and chop them finely. Fry in the bacon fat.
- Place the mushrooms in the prepared baking dish.

- Take a bowl and mix the crumbled bacon with the fried, chopped mushroom stems and the remaining ingredients. Add some of the mix to each mushroom.
- Bake for 25-30 minutes or until the mushrooms turn golden brown.

Low carb Asian cabbage stir-fry:

This is not just an easy recipe but is deliciously tasty recipe as well. This is going to be one of your favorite recipes even after your ketogenic diet days. So, take your utensils out and prepare the recipe!

Time required:

10 minutes, ready to serve in 55 minutes

Ingredients:

- o Butter – 4 oz
- o Vinegar – 1 tsp
- o Green cabbage – 1 lb.
- o Onion powder – 1 tsp
- o Minced garlic – 2 cloves
- o Chili flakes – 1 tsp
- o Chopped garlic – 2 oz
- o Ground beef or turkey – 1 ¼ lbs.
- o Sesame oil – 1 tsp
- o Salt – 1 tsp
- o Ground black pepper – ¼ tsp
- o Wasabi mayonnaise – 1 cup

Instructions:

- Shred the cabbage finely using a sharp knife or a food processor.
- Fry the cabbage in half of the butter in a large frying or wok pan on medium-high heat. It takes a while for the cabbage to soften, but don't let it turn brown.
- Add spices and vinegar. Stir and fry for a couple of minutes more. Put the cabbage in a bowl.
- Melt the rest of the butter in the same frying pan. Add garlic, chili flakes and ginger. Sauté for a few minutes.
- Add ground meat and brown until the meat is thoroughly cooked and most of the juices have evaporated. Lower the heat a little.
- Add scallions and cabbage to the meat. Stir until everything is hot. Salt and pepper to taste. Drizzle with sesame oil before serving.
- Mix together the wasabi mayonnaise by starting with a small amount of wasabi and adding more until the flavor is just right. Serve the stir-fry warm with a dollop of wasabi mayonnaise on top.

Keto Salmon with cream sauce and duck fat:

This tasty and delicious combination of salmon and cream sauce is going to blow your mind. You will not remember any other taste once you have tasted this dish. A creamy and full of fat recipe that is going to take your lunch table to another level.

Time required:

15 minutes, ready to serve in 30 minutes.

Ingredients:

- Salmon filet – 1 ½ lb.
- Dried tarragon – 1 tsp
- Dried dill weed – 1 tsp
- Duck fat – 1 tsp
- Salt and pepper to tase
- For cream sauce:
- Butter – 2 tsp
- Heavy cream – ¼ cup
- Dried tarragon – ½ tsp
- Dried dill weed – ½ tsp
- Salt and pepper to taste

Instructions:

- Slice the salmon in half and make two filets.
- Season flesh of fish with spices and skin with salt and pepper.
- Take a skillet and heat duck fat in it over medium heat. Fry the salmon filets in the duck fat for about 6 minutes until skin is crispy.

- Reduce heat and flip salmon. Then cook it for about 15 minutes until cooked thoroughly.
- Remove the fish from skillet and use the juices left in skillet for making sauce. Add brown butter and spices in the pan along with heavy cream mixture. Mix well and serve the sauce with salmon and enjoy the meal.

Ensalada De Taco:

You are going to fall in love with this unique yet delicious dish. Get ready and jump into your kitchen.

Time required:

About 25 minutes

Ingredients:

- Ground beef – 1 pound
- Taco seasoning – 1 ½ tsp
- Bell taco sauce – 2 tsp
- Chopped ice burg lettuce -12 ounces

- Diced tomato – 3 oz

- Shredded cheddar cheese – 3 oz

- Sour cream – 6 tsp

- Salsa – 6 tsp

- Guacamole – ¾ cup

Instructions:

- Brown the ground beef and drain out fat.

- Stir in seasoning mixture and taco sauce. don't make it too thick. Add a little water if consistency is too thick.

- Assemble ingredients on prepared salad. Top with your favorite toppings and serve.

Baked Chicken nuggets:

Time required:

10 minutes, ready to serve in 30 minutes

Ingredients:

- Almond flour – ¼
- Chili powder – 1 tsp
- Paprika – ½ tsp
- Boneless chicken thighs – 2 pounds
- Salt and pepper to taste
- 2 large eggs

Instructions:

- Preheat the oven to 400 degrees and line a baking sheet with parchment paper or grease it using cooking spray.
- Take a bowl and stir together almond flour, paprika and chili powder.

- o Season the chicken with salt and pepper and then dip in the beaten eggs. Then soak the chicken pieces in almond flour mixture and put on the prepared baking sheet.
- o Bake for about 20 minutes until brown and crispy. Do not let them cool, serve hot and enjoy the meal!

Taco salad with creamy dressing:

Time required:

10 minutes, ready to serve in 20 minutes

Ingredients:

- Ground beef – 6 oz
- Ground cumin – 1 tsp
- Chili powder – 1 tsp
- Chopped lettuce – 4 cups
- Diced tomatoes – ½ cup
- Diced red onion – ¼ cup
- Shredded cheddar cheese – ¼ cup
- Apple vinegar – 1 tsp
- Pinch of paprika
- Salt and pepper to taste

Instructions:

- Cook the ground beef in a skillet over medium heat until browned. Drain the fat using paper towel. Then season with salt and pepper and stir in taco seasoning.
- Fry for 5 minutes on the heat.
- Take two bowls and divide the lettuce between the two-salad bowls. Add the diced tomatoes, red onions and cheddar cheese into the bowls.
- Whisk in the remaining ingredients and drizzle over the salads to serve.

Fat bomb sandwich:

This sandwich containing bacon, lettuce, tomato and avocado is really a fat bomb. You are going to love it.

Time required:

30 minutes

Ingredients:

- o Softened cream cheese – 1 oz
- o Un cooked bacon – 2 slices
- o Sliced avocado – ¼ cup

- Tomato – 1
- Shredded lettuce – ¼ cup
- Tartar cream a pinch

Instructions:

- For the bread, Preheat the oven to 300 degrees and line a baking sheet with parchment.
- Beat the egg whites with cream of tartar and salt until soft peaks form.
- Whisk the cream cheese and egg yolk until smooth and pale yellow.
- Fold in egg whites a little at a time until well combined.
- Spoon the batter onto the baking sheet into tw even circles and bake for around 25 minutes until brown and firm.
- Cook the bacon in a skillet until crispy then drain using paper towel.
- Assemble the sandwich with bacon, avocado, lettuce and tomato.
- Your fat bomb sandwich is ready to serve, enjoy the meal!

Keto cheesy chicken salad:

A true keto salad classic: moist chicken and crispy bacon are served on a bed of crunchy Romaine lettuce. In our version, we don't skimp on the dressing or the parmesan cheese!

Time require:

15 minutes, ready to serve in 35 minutes

Ingredients:

For dressing:

- Mayonnaise – ½ cup
- Lemon zest – ½ lemon
- Shredded parmesan cheese – ¼ cup
- Chopped garlic clove
- Chopped filets of anchovies – 2 tsp

- Dijon mustard – 1 tsp
- Salt and pepper
- For salad:
- Shredded parmesan cheese – ½ cup
- Chopped lettuce – 7 oz
- Olive oil – 1 tsp
- Chicken breasts - 12 oz
- Bacon – 3 oz
- Salt and pepper to taste

Instructions:

- Preheat the oven to 350°F (175°C).
- Mix the ingredients for the dressing with a whisk or an immersion blender. Set aside in the refrigerator.
- Place the chicken breasts in a greased baking dish.
- Season the chicken with salt and pepper and drizzle olive oil or melted butter on top. Bake the chicken in the oven for about 20 minutes or until fully cooked through. You can also cook the chicken on the stove top if you prefer.
- Fry the bacon until crisp. Place lettuce as a base on two plates. Top with sliced chicken and the crispy, crumbled bacon.

- Finish with a generous dollop of dressing and a good grating of parmesan cheese.

Keto Indian butter chicken:

Butter chicken is one of our favorite Indian dishes and we know we're not the only ones! Luckily enough, we have Jill who invites you to try her keto version of this fabulous butter chicken, served with oven-roasted cauliflower.

Time required:

25 minutes, ready to serve in 1 hour 20 minutes

Ingredients:

Indian butter chicken

- 1 (4 oz.) tomato, chopped
- 1 (4 oz.) yellow onion, chopped
- ½ tbsp dried coriander (cilantro) leaves
- 2 tbsp fresh ginger
- 2 garlic cloves, chopped
- 1 tbsp tomato paste
- 1 tbsp garam masala seasoning
- ½ tbsp chili powder
- 1 tsp salt
- ¾ cup heavy whipping cream
- 2 lbs. boneless chicken thighs, cut into bite-sized pieces
- 3 oz. butter or ghee

- ½ cup fresh cilantro, for serving (optional)
- ¼ cup heavy whipping cream, for serving (optional)

Oven-roasted cauliflower

- 1 lb cauliflower, chopped into bite-sized pieces
- ½ tsp turmeric
- ½ tbsp coriander seed
- ½ tsp salt
- ¼ tsp ground black pepper
- 2 oz. butter

Instructions:

- Indian butter chicken
- Add tomato, onion, ginger, garlic, coriander, tomato paste and spices in a food processor. Mix until smooth. Add the cream and mix for a couple of seconds.
- Marinate the chicken in the mixture for at least 20 minutes, but preferably more, in the refrigerator.
- Heat a third of the butter over medium-high heat in a large frying pan. Remove the chicken from the marinade (reserve the marinade), and fry in the butter for 5 minutes.

- o Pour the marinade over the chicken and add the rest of the butter. Let simmer over medium heat for 15 minutes or until the chicken is fully cooked. Salt to taste.
- o Garnish with fresh cilantro and drizzle with a splash of cream.
- o Oven-roasted cauliflower
- o Preheat the oven to 400°F (200°C).
- o Spread the cauliflower out into an even layer in a large sheet pan.
- o Season with the spices and butter. Bake for 15 minutes.

Keto Fish casserole, creamy:

White fish swimming in a rich and creamy casserole gets kicked up a notch with the briny bite of capers and the freshness of broccoli and greens. A delicious keto dinner doesn't get any easier than this all-in-one wonder.

Time required:

10 minutes, ready to serve in 40 minutes

Ingredients:

- Small florets broccoli – 1 lb
- Scallions – 4 oz
- Small capers – 2 tsp
- Butter – 1 oz
- Heavy cream – 1 ¼ cups
- Dried parsley – 1 tsp
- Butter – 3 oz
- Dijon mustard – 1 tsp
- White fish pieces – 1 ½ lbs.
- Olive oil – 2 tsp
- Salt – 1 tsp
- Ground black pepper – ½ tsp

Instructions:

- Preheat the oven to 400°F (200°C).
- Cut the broccoli, including the stem. Peel with a sharp knife or potato peeler if the stem is rough.
- Fry broccoli in oil on medium-high for 5 minutes, until golden and soft. Season with salt and pepper.
- Add scallions, finely chopped, and the capers. Fry for another 1-2 minutes and place the vegetables in a greased baking dish.

- Nestle the fish in amongst the vegetables.
- Mix parsley, whipping cream, and mustard. Pour over the fish and vegetables. Top with slices of butter.
- Bake for 20 minutes or until the fish is cooked through, and flakes easily with a fork. Serve as is, or with a luscious green salad.

Low carb chicken garam masala:

Meet your new favorite spice blend! Garam masala makes every meal sing with earthy, aromatic, and complex flavors. Throw in silky coconut cream, sweet bell peppers and chicken, and you'll want to make this keto dish over, and over, again. And then over again!

Time required:

30 minutes, ready to serve in 50 minutes

Ingredients:

For garam masala:

- o   Ground cardamom – 1 tsp
- o   Turmeric ground – 1 tsp
- o   Ground ginger – 1 tsp
- o   Paprika powder – 1 tsp
- o   Chili powder – 1 tsp

- Ground coriander seed – 1 tsp
- Ground cumin – 1 tsp
- A pinch of ground nutmeg
- For chicken:
- Chicken breasts – 1 lb
- Diced red bell pepper – ½ oz
- Unsweetened coconut cream – 1 ¼ cups
- Chopped parsley – 1 tsp

Instructions:

- Preheat the oven to 350°F (175°C).
- Mix the spices for garam masala.
- Cut the chicken breasts lengthwise. Place a large skillet over medium high heat and fry the chicken in butter until golden brown.
- Add half the garam masala mix to the pan and stir thoroughly.
- Season with salt, and place the chicken, including the juices, in a baking dish.
- Add the finely diced bell pepper to a small bowl along with the coconut cream and remaining garam masala mix.

- o Pour over the chicken. Bake in oven for about 20 minutes.
- o Garnish with parsley and serve.

Low carb salmon butter burger:

For these salmon burgers, let's get down to the meat of the matter. They're simple to make, check. Loaded with tons of flavor, check. And they're covered with lemon butter.

Time required:

10 minutes, ready to prepare in 30 minutes

Ingredients:

For salmon burgers:

- Boneless salmon fillets – 1 ½ lbs
- 1 egg
- Yellow onion – ½
- Butter – 2 oz
- Salt and pepper – 1 tsp
- Green mash:
- Butter – 5 oz
- Broccoli – 1 lb
- Shredded parmesan cheese – ½ cup
- For lemon butter:
- Lemon juice – 2 tsp
- Butter at room temperature – 4 oz
- Salt and pepper to taste

Instructions:

Salmon burgers

- Preheat the oven to 220°F (100°C). Cut the fish into small pieces and place, along with the rest of the ingredients for the burger, in a food processor.
- Pulse for 30-45 seconds until you have a coarse mixture. Don't mix too thoroughly, this can make the burgers tough.
- Shape 6-8 burgers and fry for 4-5 minutes on each side on medium heat in a generous amount of butter or oil. Keep warm in the oven.
- Green mash
- Trim the broccoli and cut into small florets. You can use the stem as well, peel it and chop into small pieces.
- Bring a pot of lightly salted water to a boil and add the broccoli. Cook for a few minutes until soft but not until all texture is gone. Drain and discard the boiling water.
- Use an immersion blender or a food processor to mix the broccoli with butter and parmesan cheese. Season to taste with salt and pepper.

Lemon butter

- o Make the lemon butter by mixing the butter (at room temperature) with lemon juice, salt, and pepper in a small bowl using electric beaters.
- o Serve the warm burgers with a side of green mash and a melting dollop of fresh lemon butter on top.

Ketogenic cheese burger:

Heavy on the flavor and satisfaction, but light on effort!

And you don't need bread to make them wonderfully tasty

Time required:

20 minutes, ready to serve in 35 minutes

Ingredients:

For salsa:

- o Scallions – 2

- o Tomatoes – 2
- o Avocado – 1
- o Chopped cilantro – 2 tsp
- o Olive oil – 1 tsp
- o Salt a pinch

For burger:

- o Butter – 2 oz
- o Paprika powder – 2 tsp
- o Onion powder – 2 tsp
- o Garlic powder – 2 tsp
- o Shredded cheddar cheese – 1 ¾ cups
- o Ground beef – 1 ½ lb
- o Chopped oregano – 2 tsp

Toppings:

- o Dijon mustard – 4 tsp
- o Sliced dill pickles – 2 ½ oz
- o Chopped pickled jalapenos – 4 tsp
- o Mayonnaise – ¾ cup
- o Lettuce – 5 oz
- o Crumbled cooked bacon – 5 oz

Instructions:

- Chop up the salsa ingredients and stir together in a small bowl. Set aside.
- Mix in seasoning and half the cheese into the ground beef, combining with hands or a wooden spoon until blended.
- Make four burgers and fry in a pan or grill if you prefer. Season with salt and pepper, and add the remaining cheese on top towards the end.
- Serve on lettuce with mayo, bacon, pickled jalapeños, dill pickle and mustard. And don't forget the homemade salsa!

Low carb butter burger:

Traditionally, it's a Midwestern staple but we ditched the bun and made it irresistibly keto. Crispy edges, juicy bites, just perfect for the grill.

Time required:

15 minutes, ready to serve in 25 minutes

Ingredients:

- o   Butter – 1 ½ oz
- o   Ground beef or turkey – 1 lb
- o   Chopped red onion – ¼
- o   Pieces of jalapenos – 1
- o   Sliced tomatoes – 4 oz
- o   Avocado – 1
- o   Lettuce (butter head) – 1
- o   Sliced cheddar cheese – 8 slices

- Salt – 1 tsp
- Ground black pepper – ½

Instructions:

- Preheat the grill for 20 minutes on medium heat with the lid down. If you don't have a grill, you can also prepare these delicious burgers on the stovetop. Just fry the burgers in some butter in a frying pan for a few minutes on each side.
- In a bowl, combine the ground beef, salt, and pepper.
- Finely chop the onion and cut the jalapeño into small pieces. Remove the seeds first if you don't want it to be too spicy. Add onion and jalapeño to the meat and combine thoroughly with your hands.
- Form one hamburger patties per portion. First, shape them into a ball and then slowly press down. If you make them on the grill, leave them a bit thicker because they cook fast.
- Grill the patties for 5-7 minutes on each side, depending on how well done you want them. Allow them to rest for 10 minutes before serving so the juices can settle.

- While the burgers are on the grill, thinly slice the tomato. Cut the avocado lengthwise, remove the pit and spoon out the flesh.
- To assemble, take 3-4 lettuce leaves for each burger. Place burger in the middle, top each with slices of cheese and a slice of butter. Add the tomato and avocado, season with salt and pepper. Try to wrap the burger so you can easily grab it.

Keto cobb egg salad:

Egg salad is wonderful as is. But add bacon, blue cheese, avocado, and tomatoes, and you've got a lunch that you'll be dreaming about for days. The red wine vinegar–yogurt dressing is amazing and works well in regular Cobb salad, too. Deliciousness at its peak!

Time required:

15 minutes, ready to serve in 20 minutes

Ingredients:

- o Greek yogurt – 3 tsp
- o Vinegar 2 tsp
- o Mayonnaise – 3 tsp
- o Hard boiled eggs – 8
- o Cooked and crumbled bacon strips – 8
- o Sliced avocado
- o Crumbled blue cheese – ½ cup
- o Halved cherry tomatoes – ½ cup
- o Chopped chives – 2 tsp
- o Kosher salt
- o Ground black pepper

Instructions:

Take a small bowl and stir together mayonnaise, yogurt and red wine vinegar. Sprinkle salt and pepper.

Take a large bowl and gently mix eggs, bacon, avocado, blue cheese and cherry tomatoes. Slowly add mayonnaise dressing and lightly coat the ingredients. Sprinkle salt and pepper.

Then top with your favorite toppings and enjoy!

Keto buffalo shrimp lettuce wraps:

Time required:

20 minutes, ready to serve in 30 minutes

Ingredients:

- Crumbled blue cheese – ½ cup
- Sliced celery – 1 rib
- Finely chopped onion – ¼ red
- Shrimp with tails removed – 1 lb
- Olive oil – 1 tsp
- Hot sauce – ¼ cup
- Minced garlic cloves – 2
- Butter – ¼ tsp
- Kosher salt
- Ground black pepper

Instructions:

- For making buffalo sauce, take a sauce pan and melt butter in it over medium heat. Add garlic and cook for 1 minute until fragrant. Add hot sauce and stir until combined. Turn heat low while cooking shrimps.
- For making shrimp, take a skillet and heat oil in it over medium heat. Add shrimp and sprinkle salt and pepper. Cook until pink and opaque on both sides for about 2 minutes. Turn off heat and add buffalo sauce and coat the shrimps.

- Add a small scoop of shrimp to the center of a romaine leaf, then top with red onion, celery, and blue cheese.

Low carb caprese zoodles:

Time required:

10 minutes, ready to serve in 25 minutes

Ingredients:

- Zucchini – 4
- Halved cherry tomatoes- 2 cup
- Mozzarella balls – 1 cup
- Balsamic vinegar – 2 tsp
- Virgin olive oil – 2 tsp

- o Fresh basil leaves – ¼ cup
- o Kosher salt
- o Ground black pepper

Instructions:

- o Using a spiralizer, create zoodles out of zucchini.
- o Add zoodles to a large bowl, toss with olive oil and season with salt and pepper. Let marinate 15 minutes.
- o Add tomatoes, mozzarella and basil to zoodles and toss until combined.
- o Drizzle with balsamic and serve.

Broccoli salad:

Time required:

15 minutes, ready to serve in 35 minutes

Ingredients:

For salad:

- o Shredded cheddar – ½ cup
- o Sliced onion – ¼
- o Toasted sliced almonds – ¼ cup
- o Cooked bacon – 3 slices
- o Chopped chives – 2 tsp
- o Broccoli – 3 heads

For dressing:

- o Mayonnaise – 2/3 cups
- o Apple vinegar – 3 tsp
- o Dijon mustard – 1 tsp
- o Kosher salt
- o Ground black pepper

Instructions:

- o In a medium pot or saucepan, bring 6 cups of salted water to a boil. While waiting for the water to boil, prepare a large bowl with ice water.
- o Add broccoli florets to the boiling water and cook until tender, 1 to 2 minutes. Remove with a slotted spoon and place in the prepared bowl of ice water. When cool, drain florets in a colander.
- o In a medium bowl, whisk to combine dressing ingredients. Season to taste with salt and pepper.
- o Combine all salad ingredients in a large bowl and pour over dressing. Toss until ingredients are combined and fully coated in dressing. Refrigerate until ready to serve.

Ketogenic bacon sushi:

Time required:

10 minutes, ready to serve in 30 minutes

Ingredients:

- o 6 slices bacon, halved
- o 2 Persian cucumbers, thinly sliced
- o 2 medium carrots, thinly sliced
- o 1 avocado, sliced
- o 4 oz. cream cheese, softened
- o Sesame seeds, for garnish

Instructions:

- o Preheat oven to 400º. Line a baking sheet with aluminum foil and fit it with a cooling rack. Lay bacon halves in an even layer and bake until slightly crisp but still pliable, 11 to 13 minutes.
- o Meanwhile, cut cucumbers, carrots, and avocado into sections roughly the width of the bacon.
- o When bacon is cool enough to touch, spread an even layer of cream cheese on each slice. Divide vegetables evenly between the bacon and place on one end. Roll up vegetables tightly.
- o Garnish with sesame seeds and serve.

Chicken wrapped in lettuce:

Time required:

15 minutes, ready to serve in 30 minutes

Ingredients:

- o   3 tbsp. hoisin sauce
- o   2 tbsp. low-sodium soy sauce
- o   2 tbsp. rice wine vinegar

- 1 tbsp. Sriracha (optional)
- 1 tsp. sesame oil
- 1 tbsp. extra-virgin olive oil
- 1 medium onion, diced
- 2 cloves garlic, minced
- 1 tbsp. freshly grated ginger
- 1 lb. ground chicken
- 1/2 c. canned water chestnuts, drained and sliced
- 2 green onions, thinly sliced
- Kosher salt
- Freshly ground black pepper
- Large leafy lettuce (leaves separated), for serving
- Cooked white rice, for serving (optional)

Instructions:

- Make the sauce: In a small bowl, whisk together hoisin sauce, soy sauce, rice wine vinegar, Sriracha, and sesame oil.
- In a large skillet over medium-high heat, heat olive oil. Add onions and cook until soft, 5 minutes, then stir in garlic and ginger and cook until fragrant, 1 minute more. Add ground chicken and cook until

opaque and mostly cooked through, breaking up meat with a wooden spoon.

o Pour in sauce and cook 1 to 2 minutes more, until sauce reduces slightly and chicken is cooked through completely. Turn off heat and stir in chestnuts and green onions. Season with salt and pepper.

o Spoon rice, if using, and a large scoop (about 1/4 cup) of chicken mixture into center of each lettuce leaf. Serve immediately.

o Enjoy the meal!

Zucchini Sushi:

Time required:

20 minutes, ready to serve in 20 minutes

Ingredients:

- ○ Zucchini – 2 mediums
- ○ Softened cream cheese – 4 0z
- ○ Lime juice – 1 tsp
- ○ Crab meat – 1 cup
- ○ Sliced carrot – ½
- ○ Cucumber – ½
- ○ Toasted sesame seeds – 1 tsp
- ○ Avocado – ½
- ○ Sriracha hot sauce – 1 tsp

Instructions:

- o Using a vegetable peeler, slice each zucchini into thin flat strips. Place zucchini on paper towel–lined plate to sit while you prep the rest of your ingredients.
- o In a medium bowl, combine cream cheese, Sriracha, and lime juice.
- o On a cutting board, lay 2 zucchini slices down horizontally (so that the long side is facing you). Spread a thin layer of cream cheese on top, then top the left side with a pinch each of crab, carrot, avocado, and cucumber.
- o Starting from the left side, tightly roll up zucchini. Repeat with the remaining zucchini slices and fillings. Sprinkle with sesame seeds before serving.

Low carb egg roll bowls:

Time required:

10 minutes, ready to serve in 35 minutes

Ingredients:

- o 1 tbsp. vegetable oil
- o 1 clove garlic, minced
- o 1 tbsp. minced fresh ginger
- o 1 lb. ground pork
- o 1 tbsp. sesame oil
- o ½ onion, thinly sliced
- o 1 c. shredded carrot
- o ¼ green cabbage, thinly sliced
- o 1/4 c. soy sauce
- o 1 tbsp. Sriracha
- o 1 green onion, thinly sliced
- o 1 tbsp. sesame seeds

Instructions:

- o In a large skillet over medium heat, heat vegetable oil. Add garlic and ginger and cook until fragrant, 1 to 2 minutes. Add pork and cook until no pink remains.

o Push pork to the side and add sesame oil. Add onion, carrot, and cabbage. Stir to combine with meat and add soy sauce and Sriracha. Cook until cabbage is tender, 5 to 8 minutes.

o Transfer mixture to a serving dish and garnish with green onions and sesame seeds. Serve.

Keto Quesadillas:
Time required:

10 minutes, ready to serve in 35 minutes

Ingredients:

o 1 tbsp. extra-virgin olive oil

- 1 bell pepper, sliced
- ½ yellow onion, sliced
- 1/2 tsp. chili powder
- Kosher salt
- Freshly ground black pepper
- 3 c. shredded Monterey Jack
- 3 c. shredded cheddar
- 4 c. shredded chicken
- 1 avocado, thinly sliced
- 1 green onion, thinly sliced
- Sour cream, for serving

Instructions:

- Preheat oven to 400º and line two medium baking sheets with parchment paper.
- In a medium skillet over medium-high heat, heat oil. Add pepper and onion and season with chili powder, salt, and pepper. Cook until soft, 5 minutes. Transfer to a plate.
- In a medium bowl, stir together cheeses. Add 1 1/2 cups of cheese mixture into the center of both prepared baking sheets. Spread into an even layer and shape into a circle, the size of a flour tortilla.

- Bake cheeses until melty and slightly golden around the edge, 8 to 10 minutes. Add onion-pepper mixture, shredded chicken, and avocado slices to one half of each. Let cool slightly, then use the parchment paper and a small spatula to gently lift and fold one side of the cheese "tortilla" over the side with the fillings. Return to oven to heat, 3 to 4 minutes more. Repeat to make 2 more quesadillas.
- Cut each quesadilla into quarters. Garnish with green onion and sour cream before serving.

Keto dinner recipes

Keto corned beef & cabbage:

Time required:

15 minutes, ready to serve in 5 hours

Ingredients:

- o 3-4 lbs corned beef
- o 2 onions, quartered
- o 4 celery stalks, quartered crosswise

- 1 package pickling spices
- Kosher salt Black pepper
- 1 medium green cabbage, cut into 2" wedges
- 2 carrots, peeled and cut into 2" pieces
- 1/2 c. Dijon mustard
- 2 tbsp. apple cider vinegar
- 1/4 c. mayonnaise
- 2 tbsp. capers, roughly chopped, plus 1 tsp brine
- 2 tbsp. parsley, roughly chopped

Instructions:

- Place corned beef, onion, celery, and pickling spices into a large pot. Add enough water to cover by 2", season with salt and pepper, and bring to a boil. Reduce heat to low, cover, and simmer until very tender, 3–3 1/2 hours.
- Meanwhile, whisk Dijon mustard and apple cider vinegar in a small bowl and season with salt and pepper. In another bowl, mix mayo, capers, caper brine, and parsley. Season with salt and pepper
- Add cabbage and carrots and continue to simmer for 45 minutes to 1 hour more, until cabbage is tender. Remove meat, cabbage, and carrots from

pot. Slice corned beef and season with more salt and pepper.

o   Serve with both sauces on the side for dipping.

Ketogenic beef stew:

Time required:

15 minutes, ready to serve in 1 hour 45 minutes

Ingredients:

- o   2 lb. beef chuck roast, cut into 1" pieces
- o   Kosher salt
- o   Freshly ground black pepper
- o   2 tbsp. extra-virgin olive oil
- o   8 oz. Baby belle mushrooms, sliced
- o   1 small onion, chopped
- o   1 medium carrot, peeled and cut into rounds
- o   2 stalks celery, sliced
- o   3 cloves garlic, minced
- o   1 tbsp. tomato paste

- 6 c. low-sodium beef broth
- 1 tsp. fresh thyme leaves
- 1 tsp freshly chopped rosemary

Instructions:

- Pat beef dry with paper towels and season well with salt and pepper. In a large pot over medium heat, heat oil. Working in batches, add beef and sear on all sides until golden, about 3 minutes per side. Remove from pot and repeat with remaining beef, adding more oil as necessary.
- To same pot, add mushrooms and cook until golden and crispy, 5 minutes. Add onion, carrots, and celery and cook until soft, 5 minutes. Add garlic and cook until fragrant, 1 minute more. Add tomato paste and stir to coat vegetables.
- Add broth, thyme, rosemary, and beef to pot and season with salt and pepper. Bring to a boil and reduce heat to a simmer. Simmer until beef is tender, 50 minutes to an hour.

Keto low carb stuffed cabbage:

Time required:

15 minutes, ready to serve in 1 hour 45 minutes

Ingredients:

For the sauce:

- o   1 (14-oz.) can diced tomatoes
- o   1 tbsp. apple cider vinegar
- o   1/2 tsp. red pepper flakes
- o   1 tsp. onion powder
- o   1 tsp. garlic powder
- o   1 tsp. dried oregano
- o   Kosher salt Freshly ground black pepper
- o   1/4 c. extra-virgin olive oil

For the cabbage rolls:

- o   12 cabbage leaves
- o   1 lb. ground beef
- o   3/4 lb. ground pork
- o   1 c. riced cauliflower

- 3 green onions, thinly sliced
- 1/4 c. chopped parsley, plus more for serving
- Freshly ground black pepper

Instructions:

For the sauce:

- Preheat oven to 375°. Puree tomatoes, apple cider vinegar, red pepper flakes, onion powder, garlic powder, and oregano in a blender; season with salt and pepper.
- In a large deep skillet (or large pot) over medium heat, heat oil. Add pureed tomato sauce, bring to a simmer, then lower to medium-low and simmer for 20 minutes, until slightly thickened.

For the cabbage rolls:

- In a large pot of boiling water, blanch cabbage leaves until tender and flexible, about 1 minute. Set aside.
- Make filling: in a large bowl, combine ½ c. tomato sauce, ground meats, cauliflower rice, scallions, and parsley. Season with salt and pepper.

- Spread a thin layer of sauce on the bottom of a large baking dish. Using a paring knife, cut out the hard triangular rib from each cabbage leaf. Place about ⅓ cup filling into one end of each leaf, then roll up, tucking in the sides as you roll. Place rolls seam side-down on top of sauce in baking dish. Spoon remaining sauce on top of cabbage rolls. Bake 45 minutes to 55 minutes, until the meat is cooked through and internal temperature reaches 150°
- Garnish with more parsley before serving.

Ketogenic cheese and Mac:

Time required:

20 minutes, ready to serve in 1 hour 20 minutes

Ingredients:

For the Mac & Cheese

- ○ Butter, for baking dish
- ○ 2 medium heads cauliflower, cut into florets
- ○ 2 tbsp. extra-virgin olive oil
- ○ Kosher salt
- ○ 1 c. heavy cream
- ○ 6 oz. cream cheese, cut into cubes
- ○ 4 c. shredded cheddar
- ○ 2 c. shredded mozzarella
- ○ 1 tbsp. hot sauce (optional)
- ○ Freshly ground black pepper

For the topping

- ○ 4 oz. pork rinds, crushed
- ○ 1/4 c. freshly grated Parmesan
- ○ 1 tbsp. extra-virgin olive oil
- ○ 2 tbsp. freshly chopped parsley, for garnish

Instructions:

- ○ Preheat oven to 375° and butter a 9"-x-13" baking dish. In a large bowl, toss cauliflower with 2 tablespoons oil and season with salt. Spread cauliflower onto two large baking sheets and roast until tender and lightly golden, about 40 minutes.

- Meanwhile, in a large pot over medium heat, heat cream. Bring up to a simmer, then decrease heat to low and stir in cheeses until melted. Remove from heat, add hot sauce if using and season with salt and pepper, then fold in roasted cauliflower. Taste and season more if needed.
- Transfer mixture to prepared baking dish. In a medium bowl stir to combine pork rinds, Parmesan, and oil. Sprinkle mixture in an even layer over cauliflower and cheese.
- Bake until golden, 15 minutes. If desired, turn oven to broil to toast topping further, about 2 minutes.
- Garnish with parsley before serving.

Ketogenic chicken fried:

Time required:

15 minutes, ready to serve in 1 hour 15 minutes

Ingredients:

For the chicken

- o   6 bone-in, skin-on chicken breasts (about 4 lbs.)
- o   Kosher salt
- o   Freshly ground black pepper
- o   2 large eggs
- o   1/2 c. heavy cream
- o   3/4 c. almond flour
- o   1 1/2 c. finely crushed pork rinds

- 1/2 c. freshly grated Parmesan
- 1 tsp. garlic powder
- 1/2 tsp. Paprika

For the spicy mayo

- 1/2 c. mayonnaise
- 1 1/2 tsp. hot sauce

Instructions:

- Preheat oven to 400° and line a large baking sheet with parchment paper. Pat chicken dry with paper towels and season with salt and pepper.
- In a shallow bowl whisk together eggs and heavy cream. In another shallow bowl, combine almond flour, pork rinds, Parmesan, garlic powder, and paprika. Season with salt and pepper.
- Working one at a time, dip chicken in egg mixture and then in almond flour mixture, pressing to coat. Place chicken on prepared baking sheet.
- Bake until chicken is golden and internal temperature reaches 165°, about 45 minutes.

- o Meanwhile make dipping sauce: In a medium bowl, combine mayonnaise and hot sauce. Add more hot sauce depending on preferred spiciness level.
- o Serve chicken warm with dipping sauce.

Garlic rosemary chops:

Time required:

10 minutes, ready to serve in 30 minutes

Ingredients:

- o 4 pork loin chops
- o kosher salt Freshly ground black pepper
- o 1 tbsp. freshly minced rosemary
- o 2 cloves garlic, minced
- o 1/2 c. (1 stick) butter, melted
- o 1 tbsp. extra-virgin olive oil

Instructions:

- o Preheat oven to 375°. Season pork chops generously with salt and pepper.

- In a small bowl mix together butter, rosemary, and garlic. Set aside.
- In an oven safe skillet over medium-high heat, heat olive oil then adds pork chops. Sear until golden, 4 minutes, flip and cook 4 minutes more. Brush pork chops generously with garlic butter.
- Place skillet in oven and cook until cooked through (145° for medium), 10-12 minutes. Serve with more garlic butter.

Keto Ranch chicken with cheese:

Time required:

10 minutes, ready to serve in 35 minutes

Ingredients:

- o 4 slices thick-cut bacon
- o 4 boneless skinless chicken breasts (about 1 3/4 lbs.)
- o Kosher salt
- o Freshly ground black pepper
- o 2 tsp. ranch seasoning
- o 1 1/2 c. shredded mozzarella
- o Chopped chives, for garnish

Instructions:

- o In a large skillet over medium heat, cook bacon, flipping once, until crispy, about 8 minutes. Transfer to a paper towel–lined plate. Drain all but 2 tablespoons of bacon fat from the skillet.
- o Season chicken with salt and pepper. Return skillet to medium-high heat, add chicken and cook until

golden and just cooked through, about 6 minutes per side.

- o Reduce heat to medium and sprinkle chicken with ranch seasoning and top with mozzarella. Cover the skillet and cook, until cheese is melted and bubbly, about 5 minutes.
- o Crumble and sprinkle bacon and chives on top before serving.

Garlicky Lemon Mahi-Mahi:

Time required:

10 minutes, ready to serve in 30 minutes

Ingredients:

94

- 3 tbsp. butter, divided
- 2 tbsp. extra-virgin olive oil, divided
- 4 (4-oz.) mahi-mahi fillets
- Kosher salt
- Freshly ground black pepper
- 1 lb. asparagus
- 3cloves garlic, minced
- 1/4 tsp. crushed red pepper flakes
- 1lemon, sliced
- Zest and juice of 1 lemon
- 1 tbsp. freshly chopped parsley, plus more for garnish

Instructions:

- In a large skillet over medium heat, melt 1 tablespoon each of butter and olive oil. Add mahi-mahi and season with salt and pepper. Cook until golden, 4 to 5 minutes per side. Transfer to a plate.
- To skillet, add remaining 1 tablespoon oil. Add asparagus and cook until tender, 2 to 4 minutes. Season with salt and pepper and transfer to a plate.

- To skillet, add remaining 2 tablespoons butter. Once melted, add garlic and red pepper flakes and cook until fragrant, 1 minute, then stir in lemon, zest, juice, and parsley. Remove from heat, then return mahi-mahi and asparagus to skillet and spoon over sauce.
- Garnish with more parsley before serving.

Cheese steak lettuce:

Time required:

10 minutes, ready to serve in 30 minutes

Ingredients:

- 2 tbsp. vegetable oil, divided
- 1 large onion, thinly sliced
- 2 large bell peppers, thinly sliced
- 1 tsp. dried oregano

- Kosher salt
- Freshly ground black pepper
- 1 lb. skirt steak, thinly sliced
- 1 c. shredded provolone
- 8 large butterhead lettuce leaves
- 1 tbsp. freshly chopped parsley

Instructions:

- In a large skillet over medium heat, heat 1 tablespoon oil. Add onion and bell peppers and season with oregano, salt, and pepper. Cook, stirring often, until vegetables are tender, about 10 minutes. Remove peppers and onions from skillet and heat remaining oil in skillet.
- Add steak in a single layer and season with salt and pepper. Cook until steak is seared on one side, about 2 minutes. Flip and cook until the steak is seared on the second side and cooked to your liking, about 2 minutes more for medium.
- Add onion mixture back to skillet and toss to combine. Sprinkle provolone over steak and onions then cover skillet with a tight-fitting lid and cook

until the cheese has melted, about 1 minute. Remove from heat.

- o Arrange lettuce on a serving platter. Scoop steak mixture onto each piece of lettuce. Garnish with parsley and serve warm.

Keto Tuscan Butter Shrimp:

Time required:

5 minutes, ready to serve in 20 minutes.

Ingredients:

- o 2 tbsp. extra-virgin olive oil
- o 1 lb. shrimp, peeled, deveined, and tails removed
- o Kosher salt
- o Freshly ground black pepper
- o 3 tbsp. butter
- o 3 cloves garlic, minced
- o 1 1/2 c. halved cherry tomatoes
- o 3 c. baby spinach
- o 1/2 c. heavy cream
- o 1/4 c. freshly grated Parmesan

- 1/4 c. basil, thinly sliced
- Lemon wedges, for serving (optional)

Instructions:

- In a large skillet over medium-high heat, heat oil. Season shrimp all over with salt and pepper. When oil is shimmering but not smoking, add shrimp and sear until underside is golden, about 2 minutes, then flip until opaque. Remove from skillet and set aside.
- Reduce heat to medium and add butter. When butter has melted, stir in garlic and cook until fragrant, about 1 minute. Add cherry tomatoes and season with salt and pepper. Cook until tomatoes are beginning to burst then add spinach and cook until spinach is beginning to wilt.
- Stir in heavy cream, Parmesan and basil and bring mixture to a simmer. Reduce heat to low and simmer until sauce is slightly reduced, about 3 minutes.
- Return shrimp to skillet and stir to combine. Cook until shrimp is heated through, garnish with more basil and squeeze lemon on top before serving.

Low carb broiled salmon:

Time required:

10 minutes, ready to serve in 20 minutes

Ingredients:

- 4 (4-oz.) salmon fillets
- 1 tbsp. Grainy mustard
- 2 cloves garlic, finely minced
- 1 tbsp. finely minced shallots
- 2 tsp. fresh thyme leaves, chopped, plus more for garnish
- 2 tsp. fresh rosemary, chopped
- Juice of 1/2 lemon
- kosher salt
- Freshly ground black pepper
- Lemon slices, for serving

Instructions:

- Heat broiler and line a baking sheet with parchment. In a small bowl, mix together mustard, garlic, shallot, thyme, rosemary, and lemon juice and season with salt and pepper. Spread mixture all over salmon fillets and broil, 7 to 8 minutes.

o Garnish with more thyme and lemon slices and serve.

Low carb Zoodle alfredo:

Time required:

5 minutes, ready to serve in 20 minutes.

Ingredients:

- 1/2 lb. bacon, chopped
- 1 shallot, chopped
- 2 cloves garlic, minced
- 1/4 c. white wine
- 1 1/2 c. heavy cream
- 1/2 c. grated Parmesan cheese, plus more for garnish
- 1 (16 oz.) container zucchini noodles
- Kosher Salt
- Freshly ground black pepper

Instructions:

- In a large skillet over medium heat, cook bacon until crispy, 8 minutes. Drain on a paper towel-lined plate.
- Pour off all but 2 tablespoons of bacon, then add shallots. Cook until soft, about 2 minutes, then add the garlic and cook until fragrant, about 30 seconds. Add wine and cook until reduced by half.
- Add heavy cream and bring mixture to a boil. Reduce heat to low and stir in Parmesan. Cook until sauce has thickened slightly, about 2 minutes. Add zucchini noodles and toss until completely coated

in sauce. Remove from heat and stir in cooked bacon.

Stuffed peppers:

Time required:

10 minutes, ready to serve in 35 minutes

Ingredients:

- o   4 bell peppers, halved
- o   1 tbsp. vegetable oil
- o   1 large onion, sliced
- o   16 oz. cremini mushrooms, sliced
- o   Kosher salt

- Freshly ground black pepper
- 1 1/2 lb. sirloin steak, thinly sliced
- 2 tsp. Italian seasoning
- 16 slices provolone
- Freshly chopped parsley, for garnish

Instructions:

- Preheat oven to 325º. Place peppers in a large baking dish and bake until tender, 30 minutes.
- Meanwhile, in a large skillet over medium-high heat, heat oil. Add onions and mushrooms and season with salt and pepper. Cook until soft, 6 minutes. Add steak and season with more salt and pepper. Cook, stirring occasionally, 3 minutes. Stir in Italian seasoning.
- Add provolone to bottom of baked peppers and top with steak mixture. Top with another piece of provolone and broil until golden, 3 minutes.
- Garnish with parsley before serving.

Keto chicken soup:

Time required:

30 minutes, ready to serve in 1 hour

Ingredients:

- o 2 tbsp. vegetable oil
- o 1 medium onion, chopped
- o 5 cloves garlic, smashed
- o 2 piece fresh ginger, sliced
- o 1 small cauliflower, cut into florets
- o 3/4 tsp. crushed red pepper flakes
- o 1 medium carrot, peeled and thinly sliced on a bias
- o 6 c. low-sodium chicken broth
- o 1 stalk celery, thinly sliced
- o 2 boneless skinless chicken breasts
- o Freshly chopped parsley, for garnish

Instructions:

- In a large pot over medium heat, heat oil. Add onion, garlic and ginger. Cook until beginning to brown.
- Meanwhile, pulse cauliflower in a food processor until broken down into rice-sized granules. Add cauliflower to pot with onion mixture and cook over medium high heat until beginning to brown, about 8 minutes.
- Add pepper flakes, carrots, celery and chicken broth and bring to a simmer. Add chicken breasts and let cook gently until they reach an internal temperature of 165°, about 15 minutes. Remove from pan, let cool until cool enough to handle, and shred. Meanwhile, continue simmering until vegetables are tender, 3 to 5 minutes more.
- Remove ginger from pot, and add shredded chicken back to soup. Season to taste with salt and pepper, then garnish with parsley before serving.

Low carb BLT Burgers:

Time required:

25 minutes, ready to serve in 35 minutes

Ingredients:

- o 1 lb. bacon slices, halved
- o 1 lb. ground beef
- o kosher salt
- o fresh ground black pepper
- o 1/2 c. mayonnaise
- o Juice of 1/2 lemon
- o 3 tbsp. finely chopped chives
- o Butterhead lettuce, for serving
- o 2 tomatoes, sliced

Instructions:

- o Preheat oven to 400º and place a baking rack inside of a baking sheet (to help catch grease).
- o Make a bacon weave: On the baking rack, line 3 bacon halves side-by-side. Lift one end of the middle bacon slice and place a fourth bacon half on top of the side pieces and underneath the middle slice. Lay the middle slice back down.

- Next, lift the two side strips of bacon and place a 5th bacon half on top of the middle piece and underneath the sides. Lay the side slices back down.
- Finally, lift the other end of the middle slice and place a 6th slice on top of the side pieces and underneath the middle slice. Repeat to make a second weave.
- Season with pepper and bake until bacon is crispy, 25 minutes. Transfer to a paper towel-lined plate to blot grease. Let cool for at least 10 minutes.
- Meanwhile, make burgers: Preheat a grill (or grill pan) to medium-high heat. Shape ground beef into large patties and season both sides with salt and pepper. Grill until cooked to your liking, about 4 minutes per side for medium.
- Make herb mayo: In a small bowl, whisk together mayonnaise, lemon juice, and chives.
- Assemble burgers: For each burger, place a bacon weave on the bottom then spread it with some herb mayo. Top with burger, lettuce, tomato and remaining bacon weave. Serve immediately.

Ketogenic buns:

Time required:

5 minutes, ready to serve 20 minutes

Ingredients:

- 2 c. shredded mozzarella
- 4 oz. cream cheese
- 3 large eggs
- 3 c. almond flour
- 2 tsp. baking powder
- 1 tsp. kosher salt
- 4 tbsp. butter, melted
- sesame seeds Sesame
- dried parsley

Instructions:

- Preheat oven to 400° and line a baking sheet with parchment paper. In a large microwave-safe bowl, melt together mozzarella and cream cheese.
- Add eggs and stir to combine then add almond flour, baking powder and salt. Form dough into 6 balls and flatten slightly then place on prepared baking sheet.
- Brush with butter and sprinkle with sesame seeds and parsley. Bake until golden, 10-12 minutes.

Foil pack grilled Salmon:

Time required:

10 minutes, ready to serve in 20 minutes

Ingredients:

- o 20 asparagus spears, trimmed
- o 4 6-oz. skin-on salmon fillets
- o 4 tbsp. butter, divided
- o 2 lemons, sliced
- o kosher salt
- o Freshly ground black pepper

- o Torn fresh dill, for garnish

Instructions:

- o Lay two pieces of foil on a flat surface. Place five
  spears of asparagus on foil and top with a fillet of
  salmon, 1 tablespoon butter, and two slices lemon.
  Loosely wrap, then repeat with remaining
  ingredients until you have four packets total.
- o Heat grill on high. Add foil packets to grill and grill
  until salmon is cooked through and asparagus is
  tender, about 10 minutes.
- o Garnish with dill and serve.

Cauliflower wrapped in bacon:

Time required:

20 minutes, ready to serve in 1 hour 50 minutes

Ingredients:

- o 1/4 c. extra-virgin olive oil
- o 1/4 c. lemon juice
- o Kosher salt
- o 1 head cauliflower, leaves removed and stem trimmed so cauliflower lays flat, but still intact
- o 1 (10-oz.) package frozen spinach, thawed, water squeezed out and chopped
- o 2 large eggs, beaten
- o 4 green onions, thinly sliced
- o 2 cloves garlic, minced
- o 3/4 c. shredded cheddar
- o 4 oz. cream cheese, softened and cubed
- o 1/2 c. panko
- o 1/4 c. grated Parmesan

- 1 lb. thinly sliced bacon

Instructions:

- Preheat oven to 450°. Bring 8 cups water, oil, lemon juice, and 2 tablespoons salt to a boil in a large pot. Add cauliflower and bring back to a boil. Reduce to a gentle simmer and place a plate on top of the cauliflower to keep it submerged. Simmer until a knife easily inserts into the center, about 12 minutes.
- Using 2 slotted spoons or a mesh spider, transfer cauliflower to a small rimmed baking sheet. Let cool.
- Meanwhile, combine spinach, eggs, green onions, garlic, cheddar, cream cheese, panko, and Parmesan and place in a piping bag with a ¾-inch tip.
- Position cooled cauliflower stem side up on a rimmed baking sheet. Pipe filling between stalks of florets. Flip cauliflower stem side down, then lay strips of bacon, just slightly overlapping strips, over cauliflower, tucking ends of strips into bottom of cauliflower.

- Roast, rotating sheet halfway through, until golden all over, about 30 minutes.

Keto Cajun parmesan Salmon:

Time required:

25 minutes, ready to serve in 45 minutes.

Ingredients:

- 1 tbsp. extra-virgin olive oil
- 4 (4-oz.) fillets salmon (preferably wild)
- 2 tsp. Cajun seasoning, dived
- Freshly ground black pepper
- 2 tbsp. butter
- 3 cloves garlic, minced
- 1/3 c. low-sodium chicken or vegetable broth
- Juice of 1 lemon
- 1 tbsp. honey
- 1 tbsp. freshly chopped parsley, plus more for garnish
- 2 tbsp. freshly grated Parmesan
- Lemon slices, for serving

Instructions:

- In a large skillet over medium-high heat, heat oil. Season salmon with 1 teaspoon Cajun seasoning and pepper, then add to the skillet skin-side up. Cook salmon until deeply golden, about 6 minutes, then flip and cook 2 minutes more. Transfer to a plate.

- Add butter and garlic to skillet. When butter has melted, stir in broth, lemon juice, honey, remaining teaspoon Cajun seasoning, parsley, and Parmesan. Bring mixture to a simmer.
- Reduce heat to medium and add salmon back to skillet. Simmer until sauce has reduced and salmon is cooked through, 3 to 4 minutes more.
- Add lemon slices to skillet and serve.

Bacon Butternut Squash with cheese:

Time required:

10 minutes, ready to serve in 45 minutes

Ingredients:

- 2 lb. butternut squash, peeled and cut into 1" pieces
- 2 tbsp. olive oil
- 2 cloves garlic, minced

- 2 tbsp. chopped thyme
- kosher salt
- Freshly ground black pepper
- 1/2 lb. bacon, chopped
- 1 1/2 c. shredded mozzarella
- 1/2 c. freshly grated Parmesan
- Chopped fresh parsley, for garnish

Instructions:

- Preheat oven to 425°. In a large ovenproof skillet (or in a large baking dish), toss butternut squash with olive oil, garlic and thyme. Season with salt and pepper, then scatter bacon on top.
- Bake until the squash is tender and the bacon is cooked through, 20 to 25 minutes.
- Remove skillet from oven and top with mozzarella and Parmesan. Bake for another 5 to 10 minutes, or until the cheese is melty.
- Garnish with parsley and serve warm.

Ketogenic beef tenderloin:

Time required:

20 minutes, ready to serve in 1 hour 50 minutes

Ingredients:

For beef

- o 1/2 c. extra-virgin olive oil
- o 2 tbsp. balsamic vinegar
- o 2 tbsp. whole grain mustard
- o 3 sprigs fresh thyme
- o 3 sprigs fresh rosemary
- o 1 bay leaf
- o 2 cloves garlic, smashed
- o 2 tbsp. honey
- o 1 (2-lb.) beef tenderloin
- o 1 tsp. kosher salt
- o 1 tsp. freshly ground black pepper

- o 1 tsp. dried rosemary
- o 1 clove garlic, minced

For yogurt sauce

- o 1/2 c. Greek yogurt
- o 1/4 c. sour cream
- o 1 tsp. prepared horseradish
- o Juice of 1/2 lemon
- o Kosher salt

Instructions:

- o In a large bowl, mix together oil, vinegar, mustard, thyme, rosemary, bay leaf, smashed garlic, and honey. Add meat to bowl, cover with plastic wrap, and marinate in refrigerator for 1 hour or up to one day.
- o Preheat oven to 450º. Line a rimmed baking sheet with aluminum foil and fit a wire rack inside. Remove tenderloin from marinade and pat dry with paper towels. Season all over with salt, pepper, rosemary, and minced garlic, then place on rack.

- Roast until cooked to your liking, about 20 minutes for rare. Let rest 5 to 10 minutes before slicing.
- Meanwhile, make sauce: In a medium bowl, whisk together yogurt, sour cream, horseradish, and lemon juice, and season with salt.
- Slice tenderloin and serve with sauce on the side.

Low carb breaded shrimp:

Time required:

20 minutes, ready to serve in 35 minutes

Ingredients:

- o   Cooking spray
- o   6 oz. pork rinds
- o   1/4 c. grated Parmesan
- o   1 tsp. chili powder
- o   1/2 tsp. paprika
- o   1/2 tsp. garlic powder
- o   1/2 tsp. dried oregano
- o   Kosher salt
- o   2 large eggs, beaten
- o   Freshly ground black pepper
- o   1 lb. large shrimp

For the sauce + garnish

- o   1/2 c. mayonnaise (or sour cream)
- o   Juice of 1/2 lemon
- o   Dash of hot sauce

o   Freshly chopped parsley

Instructions:

o   Preheat oven to 450°. Grease a large rimmed baking sheet with cooking spray. In a food processor (or in a resealable bag using a rolling pin), crush pork rinds into fine crumbs. Transfer to a medium shallow bowl and whisk in Parmesan, spices, and herbs. Season mixture with salt and pepper.

o   Pour beaten eggs into a small shallow bowl. Dredge shrimp in eggs, letting excess drip, then coat in pork rind mixture.

o   Place breaded shrimp on prepared baking sheet in single layer. Bake until coating is crispy and shrimp is cooked through, 10 to 12 minutes.

o   Meanwhile, make sauce: In a small bowl, whisk together mayonnaise, lemon juice, and hot sauce. Garnish shrimp with parsley and serve.

Jerk Chicken:

Time required:

10 minutes, ready to serve in 2 hours 40 minutes

Ingredients:

- o 1 bunch green onions, plus more thinly sliced for garnish
- o 2 cloves garlic
- o 1 jalapeño, roughly chopped

- Juice of 1 lime
- 2 tbsp. extra-virgin olive oil
- 1 tbsp. packed brown sugar
- 1 1/2 tsp. ground allspice
- 1 tsp. dried thyme
- 1/2 tsp. ground cinnamon
- Kosher salt
- 8 pieces bone-in chicken drumsticks and thighs
- Vegetable oil, for grill

Instructions:

- In a blender, combine green onions, garlic, jalapeno, lime juice, oil, brown sugar, allspice, thyme, cinnamon, 1 teaspoon salt, and 2 tablespoons water and blend until smooth. Set aside 1/4 cup.
- Place chicken in a shallow dish and season with salt. Pour remaining marinade over chicken; toss to coat. Let marinate in fridge, turning once or twice, at least 2 hours or up to overnight.
- When ready to grill, heat grill to medium-high and oil grates. Grill chicken, turning occasionally, until chicken is charred in spots, about 10 minutes.

- Move chicken to a cooler part of the grill and brush with reserved marinade. Grill, covered, until chicken is cooked through, 10 to 15 minutes more.

Keto spinach stuffed peppers:

Time required:

15 minutes, ready to serve in 40 minutes

Ingredients:

- 4 assorted bell peppers, halved and seeded
- Extra-virgin olive oil, for drizzling
- kosher salt
- Freshly ground black pepper
- 2 c. shredded rotisserie chicken
- 1 (14-oz.) can artichoke hearts, drained and chopped
- 1 (10-oz.) package frozen spinach, thawed, well-drained, and chopped
- 6 oz. cream cheese, softened

- 1 1/2 c. shredded mozzarella, divided
- 1/2 c. grated Parmesan
- 1/4 c. sour cream
- 1/4 c. mayonnaise
- 2 cloves garlic, minced
- Chopped fresh parsley, for garnish

Instructions:

- Preheat oven to 400°. On a large, rimmed baking sheet, place bell peppers cut side-up and drizzle with olive oil, then season with salt and pepper.
- In a large bowl, add chicken, artichoke hearts, spinach, cream cheese, ½ cup mozzarella, Parmesan, sour cream, mayo, and garlic. Season with more salt and pepper and mix until well combined.
- Divide chicken mixture between pepper halves, top with remaining mozzarella, and bake until cheese is melty and peppers are tender, about 25 minutes.
- Garnish with parsley and serve.

Bacon Weave pizza cheesy:

Time required:

5 minutes, ready to serve in 40 minutes

Ingredients:

- o   12 slices thick-cut bacon
- o   1/2 c. pizza sauce
- o   1 c. shredded mozzarella
- o   1 c. sliced green bell pepper
- o   ¼ medium red onion, sliced
- o   1/4 c. sliced black olives
- o   1/4 c. grated Parmesan

Instructions:

- o   Preheat oven to 400°. Line a large baking sheet pan with parchment paper. To form a bacon weave, line six bacon slices side-by-side on the baking sheet. Lift up and fold back every other bacon slice, then lay a seventh slice on top in the center.

- Lay folded-back slices on top of seventh slice, then fold back the alternate slices. Place eighth slice on top, next to the seventh slice, weaving like you did before. Repeat this process four more times to complete the weave.
- Place an inverted, oven-proof cooling rack on top of the bacon slices. This helps them stay flat.
- Bake 23 to 25 minutes, or until bacon starts to crisp.
- Remove baking sheet from oven and pour off as much fat as you can. Carefully remove rack, then spread with pizza sauce leaving ½-inch or so for crust. Top with mozzarella, pepper, onions, olives, and Parmesan.
- Return sheet to oven and continue baking until cheese is melty, another 10 minutes.

Closing Notes

Hope you have tasted all the recipes and have made a new list of your favorite meals. It happens, after following ketogenic diet, your list of favorite meals changes. Now you have one more responsibility. Don't consider this book as just a single cook book; it can save someone's life if taken seriously. So, keep sharing as sharing is caring!

We all know that obesity and heavy weight has become a global health problem. A lot of people die of this disease

every year and others who live also face a lot of difficulties. They are not just facing physical difficulties but also psychological difficulties stand in their way. They bear criticism from people for their heavy weight. People would make fun out of them without caring for their feelings. And as a result, they become psychologically disturbed as well. And a human who is already physically disturbed, becomes psychologically disturbed then what is left in his or her life.

This is what I experienced in my life. I weighed 140 kg and I faced the similar physical and psychological problems. But instead of giving up in front of this world, I packed myself up and decided to lose weight and to show my mental strength to people around me. I decided that I will one day lose my weight and not only lose my own weight but will also become a kind of inspiration for other people suffering from same problems as well. I took a stand and I started my journey!

I want to mention one more thing that I am a professional chef. And I already knew many kinds of diets and I often tried a lot. But the results were not satisfactory in terms of health and in terms of taste as well. Who can judge taste better than a chief!

Then I happened to learn about ketogenic diet. I had much knowledge about this type of diet already but there were some myths related to this diet like it causes brain diseases, it caused people to die etc. So, I used to ignore Ketogenic diet. But then, after trying many options when nothing happened, I decided to study the one remaining option and that was "Ketogenic Diet".

I started following Ketogenic diet and as a chief prepared a lot of recipes that really helped me out more than any kind of diet and I got the best results. From 140 kg, I dropped to 80 kg after following Keto diet! You may get shocked by the results but it is my personal experience!

Ketogenic diet is basically a habit of healthy diet. You just need to leave high carbs meals and drinks and here you are in a journey towards losing your weight and enjoying your life!

The recipes that are given in this book are not just recipes, these are medicines that I used to lose weight and now I want to prescribe these medicines to my dear readers who are curious about losing weight but are not getting results so far.

Beauty of this book lies in a fact that it contains recipes that are not only healthier but are also tastier! These recipes will not taste less than any normal day diet or meal! Just try these easy recipes, satisfy your taste buds and also lose your weight!

You need not to worry about your heavy weight when you have got this cook book in your hands. You just need to go to the kitchen and bang!!

Author,
Mary Per